Five Senses

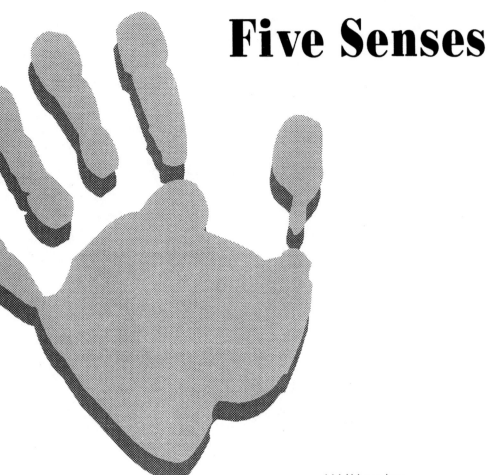

Written by
Sandra Ford Grove and Dr. Judi Hechtman

Illustrator: Catherine Yuh

Editor: Karen P. Hall

Project Director: Carolea Williams

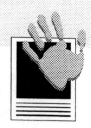

Table of Contents

Creative Teaching Press, Inc.

Introduction

The lessons in this resource have been designed to provide you with all the information you need to offer meaningful, hands-on scientific explorations with minimal preparation and maximum results. Each lesson includes the following components.

Learning Outcome

At a glance, you can see how students benefit from the activity and the knowledge they will gain.

Process Skills

The process approach to science encourages divergent thinking and provides tools for students to learn about their world. The following process skills are highlighted in student explorations.

Predicting	Defining
Observing	Inferring
Measuring	Collecting Data
Comparing	Interpreting Data
Classifying	Communicating
Experimenting	Constructing Models

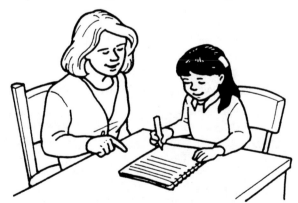

Connections

Additional activity ideas help students connect science concepts to other curriculum areas and to their own lives. This section includes a school connection to extend learning across the curriculum and a home connection to encourage family involvement.

Materials

A complete list of easy-to-find materials keeps preparation time to a minimum. You may wish to send home the parent letter (page 5) requesting help collecting materials.

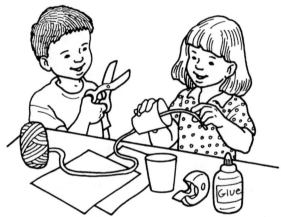

Exploration

Each exploration has been designed to challenge and teach primary students through active participation. The teacher's role is that of facilitator—providing opportunities for scientific discoveries and encouraging students to raise questions. Questioning strategies are an important tool to extend student explorations and discoveries. Each lesson includes a few suggestions to help you get started.

Conclusion

This section includes background information and expected results. It may be presented before the exploration to guide instruction or after for more open-ended discovery.

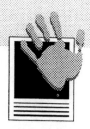

Getting Started

Classroom environment is an important part of any science unit. Following are some suggestions for creating a stimulating environment that will motivate and excite students to explore science concepts. It is equally important to encourage family involvement as you begin your unit. Suggestions for making a home connection are also included below.

Exploration Station

Designate an area in the classroom for students to explore independently. Free exploration time will help students become familiar with the materials. You may wish to include:

- optical illusions
- fragrances
- tongue map
- Braille cards
- textured materials
- eye diagram and model
- ear diagram and model
- Morse code box

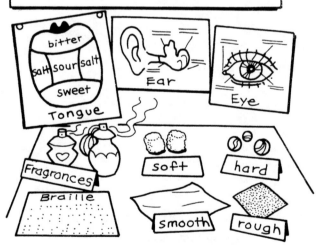

Home-School Connections

Encourage family involvement and parent communication by sending home the parent letter (page 5) at the beginning of the unit. Encourage children to share classroom activities at home and invite parents to share in their child's learning experiences.

Learning Centers

Construct independent learning centers relating to the five senses. Activities for learning centers may include examining fingerprints, observing optical illusions, decoding messages in Morse code or Braille, creating sound effects, categorizing textures, creating picture collages of the senses, and smelling fragrances.

Bulletin Board

Dedicate a bulletin board in the classroom or hallway to science work. Display student diagrams, pictures, and writings from different explorations.

Literature Connections

Collect and display books about the five senses. Use the bibliography (page 32) for book suggestions. Ask the school librarian or visit your local library for additional help. Prominently display the books in your classroom for easy access. Display poems about the five senses on classroom walls.

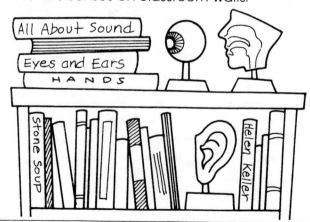

Dear Family,

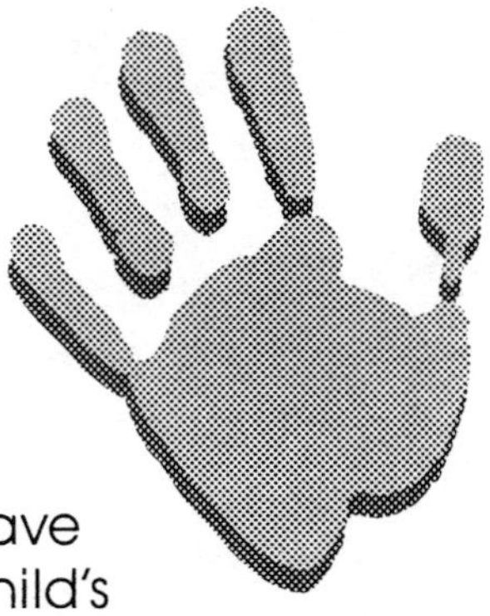

Our class is beginning an exciting science unit on the five senses. We will be exploring and investigating optical illusions, mystery sounds, touchable textures, sound vibrations, food flavors, and much more. As part of this unit, students will have assignments to complete at home. Share in your child's excitement and offer assistance whenever needed.

Some of the explorations involve materials you may have at home. If you can send any of these materials to class with your child, we would greatly appreciate it.

- film canisters
- cotton balls
- paper and Styrofoam cups
- toothpicks
- gravel
- cardboard tubes
- soup cans with both ends removed
- margarine containers

- animal magazines
- fabric scraps
- small and large cardboard boxes
- silver sequins
- kite string
- blindfolds or scarves
- nature recordings
- 2-liter soda bottles

We welcome guest speakers on subjects relating to the five senses. We would like to hear about topics such as Braille, sign language, eye care, aromatic crafts, musical instruments, and cooking. If you, or anyone you know, would like to speak to our class, please contact me.

Our study of the five senses will be fun and exciting for everyone. Thank you in advance for being a part of your child's learning experience.

Sincerely,

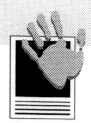

Accounting for Taste

Learning Outcome

Students discover and explore four basic tastes—sweet, salty, sour, and bitter.

Process Skills

▶ Students **predict** how foods will taste.

▶ Students **classify** food flavors as salty, sweet, sour, or bitter.

▶ Students **communicate** their results through writing and discussion.

Connections

★ School

Invite students to examine tongue cells under a microscope. Have students use cotton swabs to wipe tissue cells off their tongues and spread them onto microscope slides.

★ Home

Invite students and their families to list all food eaten during one meal and classify each item as sweet, salty, sour, bitter, or a combination of tastes.

Exploration

Divide the class into partners and distribute food items on paper plates to each pair. Discuss with students that their tongues detect four tastes. Ask students to predict in science journals the basic taste of each food item, then sample and record results—have them include where on their tongues they detect different flavors. Ask them to drink water between each sample to reduce overlap of tastes. Have students discuss and compare their predictions and results.

● Which foods taste sweet? salty? sour? bitter?
● Where on your tongue do you taste sweet flavors the strongest? salty? sour? bitter?
● In which category would you place lemonade—sweet, salty, sour, or bitter? Why is it difficult to place lemonade in only one category?

Materials

☐ salty, sweet, sour, and bitter foods (pretzels, popcorn, potato chips, gumdrops, cookies, pickles, lemon, grapefruit rind, parsley, radishes, unsweetened chocolate
☐ paper plates
☐ cups of water
☐ science journals

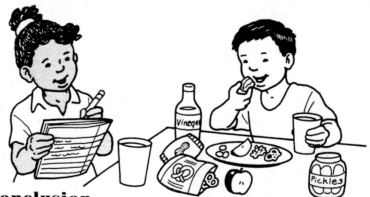

Conclusion

Your taste buds detect four basic tastes on different areas of the tongue. Sweet foods are detected on the tip of the tongue, salty foods on the sides, sour in the middle, and bitter at the back. Other flavors detected in foods are a mixture of these four main tastes. Extend learning by having students draw tongue "maps" to show where they taste sweet, salty, sour, and bitter on their tongues.

Creative Teaching Press, Inc.

The Great Taste Test

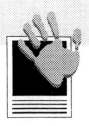

Learning Outcome

Students learn how different sweeteners affect the taste of food.

Process Skills

▶ Students **compare** the tastes of different butter samples.

▶ Students **infer** which sweeteners are in different butter samples.

▶ Students **collect data** and **communicate** their results through writing and discussion.

Connections

★ **School**

Examine different sweeteners used in prepared foods (sodas, cereals, breads, cookies). Discuss healthy substitutes for sugar products (fruit juice, apples, yogurt, raisins).

★ **Home**

Invite students and their families to conduct taste tests with different healthy snacks. Have them compare cookies made with fruit juice and natural flavors, and share their results with classmates.

Exploration

In advance, combine portions of butter with different sweeteners and store them in separate margarine containers. Label paper plate bottoms with the names of the sweeteners, spread butter samples on crackers, and place them on the appropriate plates. Provide a list of sweeteners to students and have them taste, and predict in their science journals, which sweetener was used for each sample. Have students drink water between each sample to reduce overlap of flavors. Invite students to taste small amounts of each sweetener for additional clues. After all sampling is complete, identify the sweetened butters.

● Which sweetener was easiest to identify? most difficult?

● How did artificial sweetener compare with the others?

● Which sweetener do you think tastes best? Why?

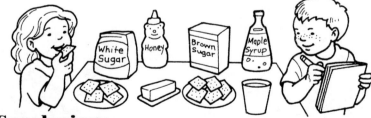

Conclusion

Various sweeteners can be added to food for flavor. Although many sweeteners taste similar (white, brown, and raw sugars), others taste quite different (honey and artificial sweetener). Artificial sweeteners are low-calorie substitutes for sugar, however, overuse may cause health problems. Extend learning by inviting students to create their own sweetened butter. Have them make butter by shaking whipping cream in baby food jars until solidified (5-10 minutes), then add different sweeteners.

Materials

☐ softened butter
☐ sweeteners (white sugar, brown sugar, raw sugar, honey, maple syrup, artificial sweetener)
☐ spoon
☐ margarine containers
☐ paper plates
☐ crackers
☐ butter knife
☐ cups of water
☐ science journals

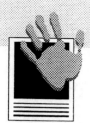

Salty or Sweet?

Learning Outcome
Students learn how spices affect food flavor.

Process Skills
▶ Students **observe** how salt affects the flavor of watermelon.

▶ Students **compare** the tastes of salted and unsalted watermelon.

▶ Students **communicate** their results through discussion.

Connections

★ School
Read aloud *The Spice Alphabet Book: Herbs, Spices, and Other Natural Flavors* by Jerry Pallotta. Have students investigate and examine spices listed in recipes and on food labels.

★ Home
Invite students and their families to prepare treats using different spices and sweeteners. Have students discuss the ingredients used and share homemade treats with classmates. Ask parents to send in their favorite recipes to create a class cookbook.

Exploration
In advance, place watermelon pieces with toothpicks on two plates. Lightly salt pieces on one plate labeled *Melon 1*. Label the plate of unsalted pieces *Melon 2*. Share and identify different spices with students and discuss how they are used to enhance food flavor. Ask students to sample and compare watermelon from each plate. Have them drink water between each taste to reduce overlap of flavors. Invite students to compare and describe how the watermelon pieces are similar and different.

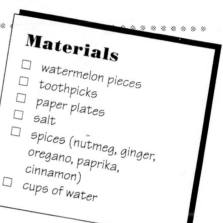

Materials
- [ ] watermelon pieces
- [ ] toothpicks
- [ ] paper plates
- [ ] salt
- [ ] spices (nutmeg, ginger, oregano, paprika, cinnamon)
- [ ] cups of water

● How is *Melon 1* similar to *Melon 2*? How are they different?
● Do you think anything was added to either melon? If so, which one?
● Why are spices added to food? What are some spices used in cooking?

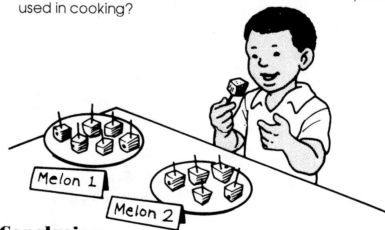

Melon 1

Melon 2

Conclusion
Spices are added to food to enhance flavor. Salt is a common spice added to many different foods. Salt added to some sweet foods makes them taste slightly sweeter. Extend learning by trying salt and other spices (cinnamon, nutmeg, ginger) on different types of sweet food (apples, bananas, pudding, cookies). Invite students to rank their favorites and graph results.

Creative Teaching Press, Inc.

Mixed Messages

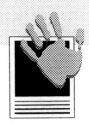

Learning Outcome

Students explore the relationship between taste and smell.

Process Skills

▶ Students taste and **predict** the identity of foods while blindfolded.

▶ Students **compare** food flavors with and without the sense of smell.

▶ Students **infer** how taste and smell work together to distinguish food flavors.

Connections

★ **School**

Explore models of the human nose. Have students use magazine pictures of different noses to create colorful collages. Invite students to write and illustrate stories about a day in the life of a nose.

★ **Home**

Invite students and their families to repeat this exploration at home. Have family members close their eyes and taste foods without using their sense of smell. Invite students to share their experiences with classmates.

Exploration

Divide the class into partners and distribute food, napkins, a blindfold, and two cups of water to each pair. Have students wear blindfolds and pinch their noses closed while partners feed them different foods. Have students drink water between each sample to reduce overlap of flavors. Ask students to guess what they're chewing and have partners record results in science journals. After sampling three or four items, have students taste the same items again without pinching their noses. After partners record results, invite them to share which foods were used. Ask students to switch roles and repeat the exploration with new foods.

● Which foods were you able to identify with your nose pinched closed?
● Do you think smelling is important for tasting food? Why?
● Why is it difficult to taste food when you have a cold or stuffy nose?

Materials
- [ ] food pieces
- [ ] napkins
- [ ] blindfolds
- [ ] cups of water
- [ ] science journals

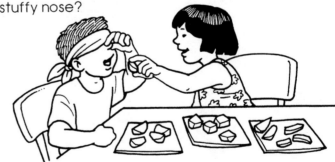

Conclusion

Smelling offers information to your brain about the taste of food. The base of the nasal cavity joins the opening to your throat to combine the sense of smell with taste. When you have a cold or stuffy nose, the sense of smell is blocked and the ability to distinguish different tastes is diminished. Extend learning by having students taste apple and potato pieces while sniffing an onion. Encourage them to discuss what happens when they send these mixed messages to the brain.

9

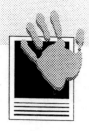

Nosy Animals

Learning Outcome

Students learn ways different animals use their noses.

Process Skills

▶ Students **compare** the size, shape, and function of different animal noses.

▶ Students **classify** ways animals use their sense of smell.

▶ Students **communicate** their knowledge through discussion and writing.

Connections

★ School

View various animal videos (such as those produced by National Geographic), and invite students to identify and describe different animal noses.

★ Home

Invite students and their families to visit zoos, farms, and nature museums to investigate and compare different animal noses.

Exploration

Distribute a lab sheet to each student. Discuss the size and shape of different animal noses and have students describe similarities and differences among their pictures. Brainstorm with students ways animals use their noses—smelling food, breathing, detecting enemies, lifting objects, burrowing, and exploring high and low places. Invite students to create their own animal noses using craft items. Have them decorate cardboard tubes, paper cups, and egg carton cups to match their favorite animal nose. Attach an elastic cord to each nose and invite students to model them for classmates.

● How is a human nose different from a horse nose? an elephant nose (trunk)? How are they similar?

● What are some ways animals use their noses?

● What would be best about having a nose like an elephant? a pig? a mouse?

Materials

☐ lab sheet (page 11)
☐ craft items (construction paper, paper cups, cardboard tubes, egg cartons, pipe cleaners)
☐ scissors
☐ glue
☐ crayons or markers
☐ elastic cords

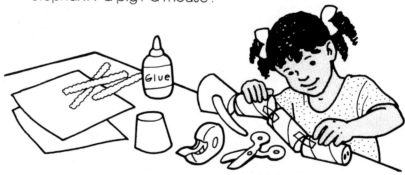

Conclusion

Most mammals rely heavily on their sense of smell to find food, detect enemies, and communicate with other members of their species. Many mammals, such as dogs and cats, use odors to identify and protect property. Compared to many animals, our sense of smell is poor, although the average person can detect more than 4,000 different scents. Extend learning by inviting partners to write and dramatize animal stories using their animal noses.

Creative Teaching Press, Inc.

Nosy Animals

How are these animal noses similar? How are they different?

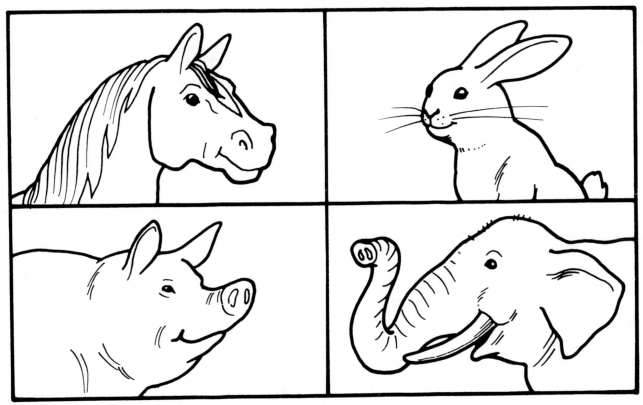

Similar: _____

_____

Different: _____

_____

Which of these animal masks can you make? What other animal noses can you create with craft items?

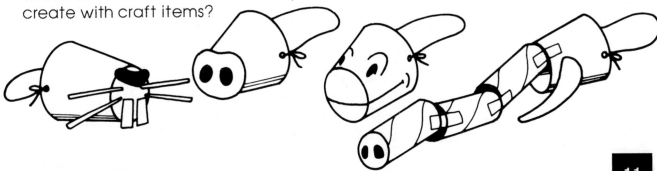

Creative Teaching Press, Inc.

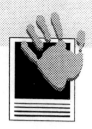

What Your Nose Knows

Learning Outcome

Students learn to recognize and sequence items using their sense of smell.

Process Skills

▶ Students **experiment** with food recognition using their sense of smell.

▶ Students **compare** and **interpret** foods in sequence using aromatic cues.

▶ Students **communicate** their results through discussion and writing.

Connections

★ School

Invite students to create scratch-and-sniff pictures. Have them brush a thin film of glue over a picture, sprinkle it with powdered juice mix or dry flavored gelatin, and let dry. Invite students to share their scratch-and-sniff pictures with classmates.

★ Home

Invite parents to cook mystery foods and have students identify the foods using their sense of smell—have students stand in different rooms of their homes to detect and identify food aromas.

Exploration

Divide the class into partners and give each pair 4-6 food pieces, index cards, and a blindfold. Ask students to color pictures and write words on index cards to match food items. Have one student from each pair wear a blindfold while partners give them food items to smell—ask partners to record food order in their science journals. Ask students to remove their blindfolds and arrange matching index cards in the order food items were smelled. Have students check and record results in their science journals, then ask partners to switch roles and repeat testing.

● Which food items were easy to identify? Which ones were difficult?

● Were you able to sequence food cards correctly? Why or why not?

● How would you know if someone was baking cookies in the kitchen if you were reading in your bedroom?

Materials

☐ food pieces (onion, pickle, lemon, peppermint, peanut)
☐ 3" x 5" index cards
☐ blindfolds
☐ crayons or markers
☐ science journals

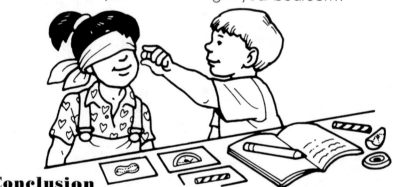

Conclusion

Scientists believe that all scents are one or a combination of seven basic smells—flowery, decay, peppermint, musk, ether, mothballs, and spicy. Most people can recognize about 4,000 different scents, however some individuals, such as a chef or a perfume maker, may be able to detect up to 10,000 different scents. Extend learning by having students sequence cards by both smelling and feeling food items. Invite students to discuss how combining senses affects their results.

12

Are You My Mother?

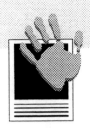

Learning Outcome

Students discover how animals use scent to recognize their young.

Process Skills

▶ Students **compare** and match different fragrances.

▶ Students **predict** the identity of mystery scents.

▶ Students **infer** how animals use scent to recognize their young.

Connections

★ School

Invite students to create aromatic books using different scented items (potpourri, dried flowers, perfumed cloth scraps, herbs). Have students write sentences to describe each aromatic scent.

★ Home

Invite students and their families to create pomander balls by covering oranges with cloves, inserting the pointed ends into the rind. Add ribbon as a final touch and hang as beautiful, aromatic ornaments.

Exploration

In advance, number the bottoms of fragrance bottles using masking tape and a permanent marker. You will need a different fragrance for each pair of students. Soak cotton balls in each fragrance and place them inside separate film canisters. Number each canister to match the numbered fragrance. Place the lids on the canisters, shake, and let them sit for at least one hour before the exploration. Separate the lids from the canisters and randomly distribute them to students. Designate the students with canister bottoms as "parents" and students with lids as "babies." Have parents and babies stand at opposite sides of the classroom, and ask students to find their partners by matching odors. Once students find their match, have them guess which fragrance was used, then check the bottles to see if they are correct.

● How were you able to find your "parent"/"baby"?
● Which fragrances smelled similar? different?
● How do you think animals identify their young?

Materials

- ☐ masking tape
- ☐ permanent marker
- ☐ fragrant items (perfumes, vanilla, almond extract, peppermint extract, pickle juice, lemon juice, cinnamon oil, vinegar)
- ☐ cotton balls
- ☐ film canisters with lids

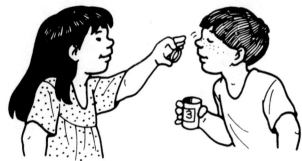

Conclusion

Animals have their own distinct scent which can be used for identification. Animal parents identify their offspring by odor, distinguishing them from other babies that may look exactly alike. Extend learning by investigating how animals use odor to track food, defend territory, and attract mates.

13

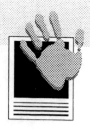

Do You Hear What I Hear?

Learning Outcome
Students learn to identify objects by sound.

Process Skills
▶ Students **observe** sounds of different objects.

▶ Students **compare** sounds of different objects.

▶ Students **infer** what an object is by listening to the sound it makes.

Connections

★ *School*
Explore and teach students Morse code. Set up a center with a Morse code chart or teach students a few letters every day. Divide the class into partners and invite students to send secret messages or practice spelling words in Morse code.

★ *Home*
Invite students and their families to create mystery noise tapes. Ask students to record sounds around the home (washers, refrigerators, vacuum cleaners, sprinklers, toilets) and have their class-mates identify the object matching each sound.

Exploration
Cover test items and have students sit with their backs toward you. Create sounds with each object, and ask students to record in their journals the identity of each "mystery" sound. After hearing all objects, have students face forward and share their predictions. Reveal the identity of each object and compare with student guesses. Have students discover and explore noises made with common household objects (rice-filled coffee cans, cellophane, metal spoons). Have partners use sound effects to create spooky stories to share with classmates.
● Which objects were easiest to recognize by sound? the most difficult?
● Which objects sound similar? different? In what way?
● How do you think blind people identify objects?

Materials
☐ test objects (baby rattle, maracas, radio, bell, ball, wristwatch alarm, whistle, electric can opener, jump rope, stapler, electronic game)
☐ household items (rice, dried beans, coffee cans, plastic bottles, cellophane, paper, foil, metal spoons, sandpaper, chopsticks)
☐ science journals

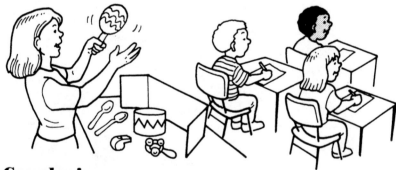

Conclusion
People often identify an object by sound. Sound consists of invisible vibrations that travel in waves. Sound waves enter the ear where they are changed into nerve signals and sent to the brain for identification. Extend learning by having students listen to and repeat clapping patterns. First have students watch, listen, and repeat patterns. Then have students close their eyes and repeat patterns by listening only.

Creative Teaching Press, Inc.

Party Lines

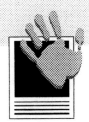

Learning Outcome

Students learn how sound vibrations travel through telephone lines.

Process Skills

▶ Students **construct models** of telephones.

▶ Students **communicate** through telephone models.

▶ Students **infer** how real telephones work.

Connections

★ School

Create a telephone center for students to explore and use during dramatic play. Discuss phone etiquette, and invite students to dramatize calls from family members, friends, movie stars, and cartoon characters. Bring in an old disassembled telephone and invite students to explore the parts.

★ Home

Invite students and their families to experiment with different containers and strings to construct telephone models at home. Invite students to share their creations with classmates.

Exploration

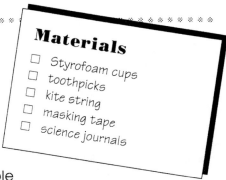

Divide the class into partners and distribute two cups, two toothpicks, six feet of string, and masking tape to each pair. Ask students to poke a small hole with a toothpick in the bottom of each cup, then thread the ends of the string through the holes. Have students secure string in place by tying each end around a toothpick or by placing tape over each hole. Ask each partner to hold one end of the "phone line" and move apart from each other until the string is straight and taut. Have one partner listen while the other speaks into his or her cup. Ask students to record in science journals messages heard, then have students switch roles.

● What happens when your partner speaks softly into the "telephone"? loudly?

● What happens when you and your partner speak into the "telephone" at the same time? Why?

● How do you think your "telephone" works?

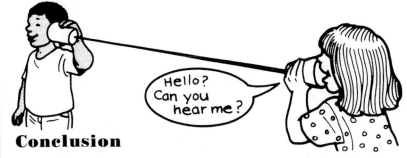

Hello? Can you hear me?

Conclusion

A telephone is an instrument that sends and receives sound from a distance by means of electricity. A person's voice enters the telephone mouthpiece, creating sound waves that are carried by an electric current to the telephone earpiece of the person at the receiving end. String "telephone" lines simulate how real telephones work—sound vibrations travel through the string and into the cup at the receiving end. Extend learning by having students create "party lines." Loop two phone lines together at the middle so student pairs are standing perpendicular to each other in a four-way conversation.

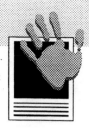

Sound Radar

Learning Outcome

Students discover that two ears detect the direction of sound better than one.

Process Skills

▶ Students **observe** and locate the direction of sounds.

▶ Students listen to and **compare** sounds using one ear versus both ears.

▶ Students **collect data** and **communicate** test results through writing and discussion.

Connections

★ **School**
Investigate and explore facts about the deaf community. Teach students the alphabet in sign language and have them practice signing words to partners.

★ **Home**
Invite students and their families to play *Hide and Seek* while blindfolded. Have students find their way by listening and following the voice of a family member.

Exploration

Tell students they are going to test whether two ears detect the direction of sound better than one.

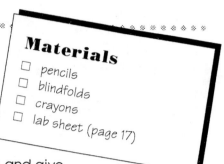

Materials
☐ pencils
☐ blindfolds
☐ crayons
☐ lab sheet (page 17)

Divide the class into partners and give each pair a blindfold, two pencils, crayons, and two lab sheets. Ask students to put blindfolds on their partners and sit them in a chair. Ask each "tapper" to record on the top half of the lab sheet the sequence and location of 4–6 taps he or she will make—if tap one is to the right of his or her partner, the tapper writes *1* on the right side of the lab sheet; if tap two is to the left, then a *2* is written to the left. Have students tap pencils together at different locations around the chair while blindfolded partners indicate by pointing from which direction they hear each tap. As each tap is made, ask students to number with crayons where the tap is heard. Have students repeat and record testing with blindfolded partners placing their thumb in one ear. Ask partners to remove blindfolds and check results. Invite students to switch roles.

● Was it easier to detect the direction of sounds using one ear or two?
● Which taps were most difficult to detect?
● Do you think it's harder to determine the location of taps far away? in noisy places? Why?

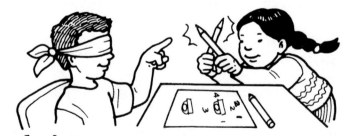

Conclusion

Using two ears helps us determine from which direction sound is coming. Taps are readily determined when they are to your right or left. It is much more difficult to determine the direction of sound when it is directly behind you because it reaches both ears at the same time. Extend learning by having students detect taps near and far away.

Creative Teaching Press, Inc.

Sound Radar

Use a pencil to number around the pictures where each tap is to be made. While testing your partner, number with a crayon where he or she hears the taps.

Testing with Both Ears

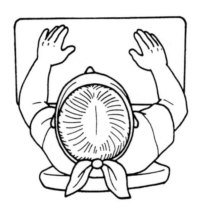

Testing with One Ear Covered

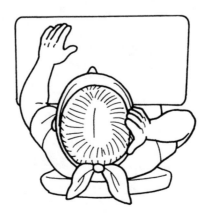

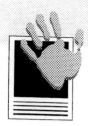

Sound Vibrations

Learning Outcome

Students discover that sound travels in waves.

Process Skills

▶ Students **construct models** of oscilloscopes to view sound waves.

▶ Students **observe** and **compare** the intensity of sound waves.

▶ Students **communicate** their results through discussion.

Connections

★ School

Investigate the structure of ears in various animals. Have students compare hearing mechanisms found in frogs, bats, crickets, and fish.

★ Home

Invite students to experiment with their oscilloscopes at home. Have them compare sound waves created by different family members.

Exploration

In advance, cover can rims with tape to protect from sharp edges. Discuss with students how we hear noises through vibrating sound waves. Tell students they will make special instruments called oscilloscopes to "see" sound waves. Distribute a can, balloon, rubber band, sequin disk, scissors, glue, and flashlight to each pair of students. Ask them to cut off balloon necks, stretch the remaining piece over one end of the can, and secure it with a rubber band. Ask students to glue a sequin disk in the center of the balloon, then face the can toward a classroom wall. Darken the room and have students shine flashlights on the disks while partners speak into the other end of the can. Ask students to observe and compare sound waves illuminated on the wall.

● What happens to the reflected light when you speak into the can?
● What happens when you speak loudly into the can? softly?
● What happens when you speak into the can with a high voice? low voice?

Materials

☐ soup cans (both ends cut off)
☐ tape
☐ round balloons
☐ rubber bands
☐ silver sequins
☐ scissors
☐ glue
☐ flashlights

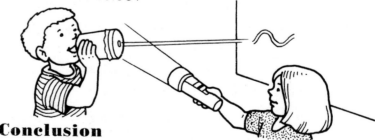

Conclusion

Loud sounds display large wave patterns through oscilloscopes; soft sounds display small ones. When high-pitched sounds project through the can, sound waves vibrate quickly; low-pitched sound waves vibrate slowly. Extend learning by inviting students to trace illuminated sound waves on butcher paper, or "feel" sound vibrations by touching their throats as they hum, cough, and growl.

Now You See It, Now You Don't

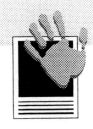

Learning Outcome

Students discover their range of peripheral vision.

Process Skills

▶ Students **experiment** with their peripheral vision.

▶ Students **collect data** to determine their range of peripheral vision.

▶ Students **compare** peripheral vision in their right and left eyes.

Connections

★ School

Invite students to make glasses that block peripheral vision. Cut empty cardboard tubes in half, add pipe cleaner bridges, and two pipe cleaner earpieces. Have students wear glasses to perform routine tasks, then share their experiences with classmates.

★ Home

Have students and their families test peripheral vision at home. Have students sit in a chalk circle and look straight ahead while parents roll a ball from different parts of the circle. Invite students to use their peripheral vision to stop the oncoming ball.

Exploration

Discuss how we use peripheral vision to view objects from the corners of our eyes. Divide the class into partners and distribute construction paper, scissors, and stickers to each pair. Have students cut out large colored triangles, squares, circles, and diamonds. Ask one student from each pair to sit in a chair, looking straight ahead, while partners slowly bring a colored shape around the chair—from the back, to the right side, and in front of the student. Have partners stop when students can identify both the color and the shape of the paper without rotating their eyes or turning their heads. Ask partners to place stickers on the floor at the point where the paper stopped. Test the left side, then have partners switch roles.

● Which were you able to identify first, the color or shape of the paper?

● Is your peripheral vision better with your right or left eye? How do you know?

● Why is peripheral vision important?

Materials
- [ ] construction paper
- [ ] scissors
- [ ] stickers

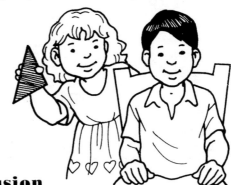

Conclusion

The retina of the eye provides us with peripheral vision. We use peripheral vision when performing such tasks as walking across a busy intersection or playing sports. Peripheral vision enables us to see objects approaching from the sides; however, we can often only distinguish color and blurred images until the object moves directly in front of us. Extend learning by having students test peripheral vision with different classroom objects or by reading word cards.

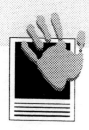

Two Eyes Are Better Than One

Learning Outcome

Students discover how their eyes work together to judge depth and distance.

Process Skills

▶ Students **experiment** and **compare** depth perception using one and two eyes.

▶ Students **collect data** to support their hypotheses.

▶ Students **communicate** their results through writing and discussion.

Connections

★ School

Invite students to test depth perception using clay balls and paper targets. Have one student from each pair stand from a distance and direct his or her partner, standing by the target, where to drop the ball. Write point values on target areas and have students calculate scores after each round.

★ Home

Invite students and their families to play a game such as horseshoes or croquet while wearing an eye patch. Have students share their results with classmates.

Exploration

Tell students they will test depth perception—the ability to see and judge distance—using both eyes versus one eye. Divide the class into partners and give each pair a ping pong ball. Have partners stand about four feet apart and toss the ball back and fourth. After ten tosses, ask one student from each pair to put on an eye patch and tally in their science journals the number of times they catch the next ten tosses. Ask them to repeat the process, this time moving two steps further apart. Have students record their results and switch roles.

● Was it easier catching the ball with both eyes uncovered or with one eye covered?

● Was it easier to catch the ball standing closer to your partner or farther away? Why?

● What would happen if you could only see out of one eye? What would you have difficulty doing?

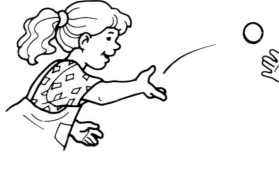

Conclusion

Depth perception is the ability to judge distance and size of objects. Because our eyes are set slightly apart, they see objects from slightly different angles. Our brain requires both perspectives to determine distance and depth accurately. Extend learning by having partners test depth perception using pencils. Have one student from each pair hold two pencils at different distances—one close to his or her body and one far away. Ask students to move pencils together until partners, standing four feet away, indicate pencils are aligned side-by-side.

Optical Illusions

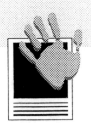

Learning Outcome

Students explore how the brain is fooled by optical illusions.

Process Skills

▶ Students **experiment** with different optical illusions.

▶ Students **compare** their initial observations with final results.

▶ Students **communicate** their results through writing and discussion.

Connections

★ **School**

Discuss how magicians use illusions for their tricks. Invite students to share magic tricks with classmates.

★ **Home**

Invite students and their families to visit local libraries and bookstores to discover more optical illusions to share with classmates.

Exploration

Distribute rulers to students and have them follow directions on the lab sheet to experiment with different optical illusions. Have students predict and compare the height of the bears, check for curvature of the square, and "fix" the broken train track. Invite students to cut out the bird and cage pictures at the bottom of the lab sheet to create their own optical illusion. Have them color, cut out, and paste each picture to the center of an index card, then paste cards back-to-back with a long piece of string in between. Ask students to observe what happens to the bird when they twirl the cards with the string.

● How were the results of the optical illusions surprising?
● What appears to happen when you twirl the bird and cage cards with the string?
● What are optical illusions? How do you think they work?

Materials

☐ rulers
☐ lab sheet (page 22)
☐ scissors
☐ index cards
☐ glue
☐ string
☐ crayons or markers

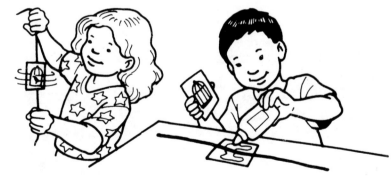

Conclusion

Although the bears appear different in height and the sides of the square seem curved, they are not. The reasons for optical illusions are not clearly understood, though some scientists believe illusions occur when our brains form preconceived images based on life experience. Extend learning by inviting students to make and explore other optical illusions. Have students repeat the twirling card activity by drawing other pairs of pictures such as a fish and fishbowl.

Creative Teaching Press, Inc.

Optical Illusions

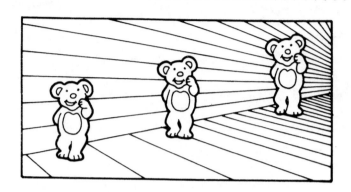

Look at the teddy bears.
Circle which one looks tallest.

Check with a ruler.
Which one is tallest? _____

Look at the square.
Are the sides straight or curved?

_____

Check with a ruler.
Are the sides straight or curved?

_____

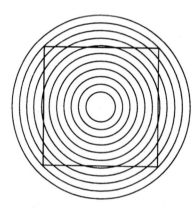

Oh no! The train track is broken and there is a train coming! But you can fix it—simply bring your nose closer to the gap and see what happens.

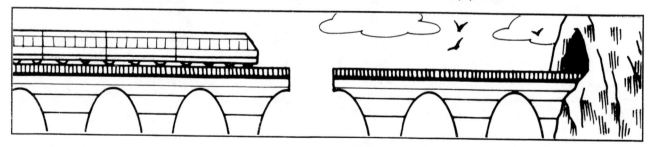

Create your own optical illusion using the bird and cage pictures, index cards, and a piece of string. Glue the pictures to index cards, and then glue the card backs together with the string in between. Twirl the cards and see what happens.

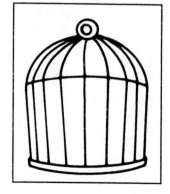
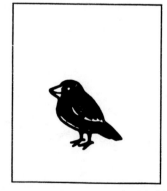

Feeling the Groove

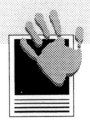

Learning Outcome

Students discover how touch can be used to identify objects.

Process Skills

▶ Students **infer** the identity of hidden objects using three of their senses.

▶ Students **collect data** and record their findings in science journals.

▶ Students **interpret** and **communicate** their results through discussion and writing.

Connections

★ School

Invite students to feel and compare objects from nature. Have students compare textures of leaves, flowers, grass, pine cones, and tree bark. Invite students to create crayon rubbings using leaves and white paper.

★ Home

Invite students and their families to feel and identify household objects while blindfolded. Have students feel their way from one room of their homes to another. Invite students to share results with classmates.

Exploration

Ask each student to secretly find and place a small classroom object inside his or her paper bag. Divide the class into pairs and have partners switch bags. First, have students shake the bags to guess the contents, then record their observations in science journals. Second, have them smell the bags and record any further clues they discover. Third, ask students to touch the outside of the bags to feel the hidden objects. Finally, have them reach inside the bags and hold the objects while closing their eyes. Ask students to record their final observations and predict the identity of the objects. Invite them to look inside the bags to check their predictions.

● What clues did you discover while shaking the bag? smelling the bag?
● What did the object feel like from the outside of the bag? How did it feel differently inside the bag?
● How does the sense of touch help you identify objects you cannot see?

Materials

☐ paper lunch bags
☐ small classroom objects (crayon, paper clip, ruler, bell, chalk, hole punch, eraser)
☐ science journals

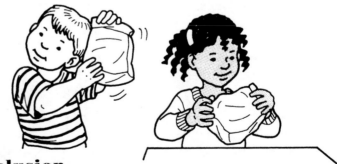

Conclusion

Smelling, hearing, and touching help you identify objects you cannot see. Certain objects have distinctive odors while others have recognizable sounds. Touching an object offers clues about texture, size, and shape. When both sight and touch are blocked, it is much more difficult to identify objects. Extend learning by having students bring mystery objects from home and repeat testing with a new partner.

Creative Teaching Press, Inc.

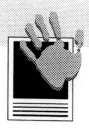

Touching Textures

Learning Outcome

Students learn to identify different textures through the sense of touch.

Process Skills

▶ Students **experiment** with textured name plates.

▶ Students feel and **compare** letters from textured name plates.

▶ Students **communicate** their results through writing and artwork.

Connections

★ School

Invite partners to explore textures around the school while blindfolded. Have partners guide blindfolded students as they feel different objects. Invite students to write about their experiences in science journals.

★ Home

Invite students and their families to explore different textures in their homes. Have students create textured animal pictures using household materials (cotton for rabbits, feathers and birdseed for birds, black and white dried beans for zebras).

Exploration

In advance, cut poster board into 4" x 8" pieces and give one to each student. Have them create textured name plates by writing their names in large print and gluing different textured materials to each letter. Collect finished name plates and divide the class into partners. Ask one student from each pair to close his or her eyes before receiving a name plate. Have students feel and identify different parts of the name plates while partners record findings in science journals. Ask students to identify which materials were used, what letters were formed, and what name was spelled. After the exploration, have students open their eyes and check their findings. Ask partners to switch roles and repeat testing.

● Were you able to "read" the name on the name plate without using your eyes? How?

● How would you describe the different textures? How does cotton compare to sand? dried beans?

● Why is the sense of touch important? How does it help identify objects?

Materials

☐ poster board
☐ scissors
☐ crayons or markers
☐ textured materials (foil, cloth strips, sand, cotton, cereal, sand, cotton, cereal, seeds macaroni, rice, marshmallows)
☐ glue
☐ science journals

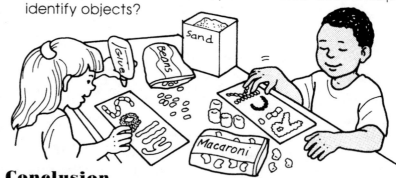

Conclusion

The sense of touch allows us to identify the size, shape, and texture of different objects. Nerve endings in our fingertips enable us to detect soft, smooth, rough, hard, and sharp textures. Extend learning by inviting students to write textured secret messages for partners to decode. Create a colorful textured bulletin board for students to enjoy.

Creative Teaching Press, Inc.

Size It Up

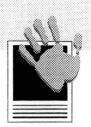

Learning Outcome

Students learn how touch can be used to distinguish height, size, and weight of objects.

Process Skills

▶ Students **compare** and **classify** objects according to height, size, and weight.

▶ Students **collect data** and record results in science journals.

▶ Students **communicate** their results through writing and discussion.

Connections

★ **School**

Invite students to determine which parts of their bodies are more sensitive to touch. Have students close their eyes while partners gently touch different body areas with a cotton swab (palm of hand, elbow, fingertip, back, thigh, knee).

★ **Home**

Invite students and their families to repeat the exploration at home using canned foods. Have students wear blindfolds and arrange cans by size, height, and weight.

Exploration

In advance, cut cardboard tubes to different heights, place objects of various weight in margarine containers, and fill 2-liter soda bottles with different amounts of water. Organize six exploration stations:

● *Station 1*—cardboard tubes numbered from shortest to tallest.

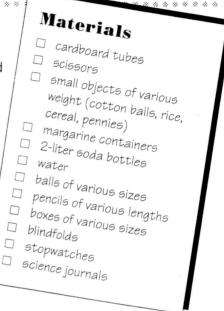

Materials

- ☐ cardboard tubes
- ☐ scissors
- ☐ small objects of various weight (cotton balls, rice, cereal, pennies)
- ☐ margarine containers
- ☐ 2-liter soda bottles
- ☐ water
- ☐ balls of various sizes
- ☐ pencils of various lengths
- ☐ boxes of various sizes
- ☐ blindfolds
- ☐ stopwatches
- ☐ science journals

● *Station 2*—balls numbered from smallest to largest.

● *Station 3*—margarine containers numbered from lightest to heaviest.

● *Station 4*—pencils numbered from shortest to longest.

● *Station 5*—boxes numbered from smallest to largest.

● *Station 6*—water bottles numbered from lightest to heaviest.

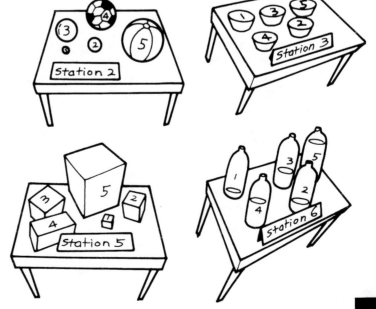

Creative Teaching Press, Inc.

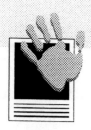

Size It Up

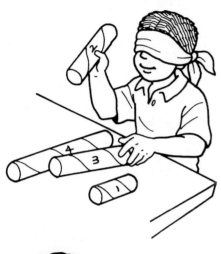

Divide the class into threes and assign a "recorder," "timer," and "test taker" for each group. Ask test takers at each station to wear blindfolds and sequence objects from smallest to largest or lightest to heaviest. Have recorders write results (number sequence) in science journals while timers use stopwatches to monitor elapsed time. Have students switch roles after each test and change stations after all group members take a turn.

- Which objects were the hardest to sequence? Which were easiest? Why?
- How did your sense of touch help you arrange objects at each station?
- Which senses combined with touch were helpful in arranging objects? How?

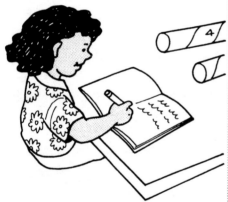

Conclusion

The sense of touch is very important. Skin contains a variety of nerve endings that detect heat, cold, pressure, and pain. Our fingers, mouths, and toes are more sensitive than other areas of our bodies since we use them more often to explore the world around us. Our sense of touch helps determine the size, weight, and height of different objects. In combination with other senses (hearing, smelling, seeing, tasting), object recognition is easier. Extend learning by having students repeat testing without blindfolds. Have them compare results and discuss how combining senses quickens and sharpens response.

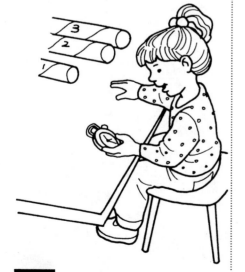

Dot-to-Dot: Learning Braille

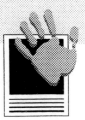

Learning Outcome

Students learn about Braille and the ability to communicate through touch.

Process Skills

▶ Students **experiment** with the Braille alphabet.

▶ Students **compare** reading Braille with written words.

▶ Students **communicate** and **interpret** data through the sense of touch.

Connections

★ School

Explore lifestyles of the blind. Read aloud *My Hands, My World* by Catherine Brighton. Invite students to imagine what it would be like to be blind and share their thoughts through writing and discussion.

★ Home

Invite students to share the Braille alphabet with their families. Have students create secret messages in Braille for family members to decode.

Exploration

Brainstorm with students different ways to communicate (spoken words, written words, body language). Write a message on the chalkboard and have students copy and read the message. Ask students to close their eyes and try repeating the process. Discuss the impossibility of reading print without vision. Distribute a pushpin, piece of cardboard, and lab sheet to each student. Introduce the Braille alphabet—explain that it is a special language of raised dots used by the blind to read and write. Have students place the lab sheet face down on cardboard and use a pushpin to poke holes through each dot in the pattern. Ask students to turn the lab sheet face up, close their eyes, and read the Braille alphabet with their fingertips.

● What is the maximum number of dots used to make a Braille letter?

● How are the Braille letters *b* and *c* similar? different? What other letters have similar dot patterns?

● How do you think blind individuals read and write words?

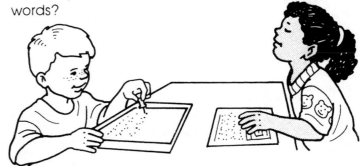

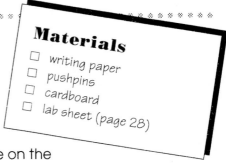

Materials
- ☐ writing paper
- ☐ pushpins
- ☐ cardboard
- ☐ lab sheet *(page 28)*

Conclusion

Blind people often compensate for lack of sight by developing a keener sense of touch, smell, and hearing. Many learn to read by touch using Braille. Some blind people can read more than 100 words of Braille a minute. Extend learning by inviting students to write words in Braille by poking letter patterns side-by-side. For added fun, have students poke holes through the back of the lab sheet maze, then feel their way from beginning to end.

Creative Teaching Press, Inc.

Dot-to-Dot: Learning Braille

A B C D E F G H I

J K L M N O P Q R

S T U V W X Y Z

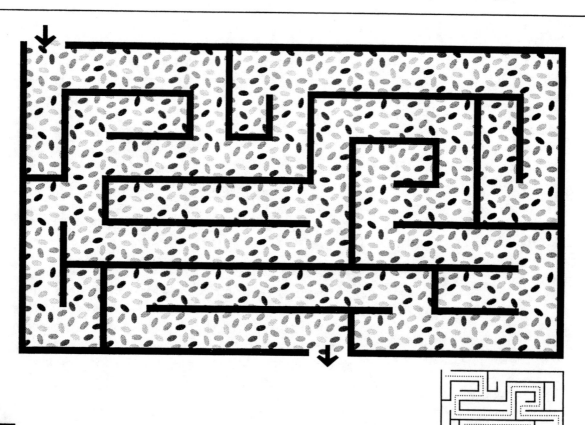

Creative Teaching Press, Inc.

Real-Life Connections

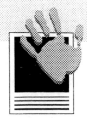

As each science topic is studied, make real-life connections to professional, community, and family life:

▶ Invite members of the medical community to speak to students about sense organs.

▶ Invite a blind or deaf individual to share his or her experiences with the class. Set up a pen-pal program with a school for the deaf or blind to encourage further awareness and communication.

▶ Invite artists, musicians, and chefs to share their creations with the class.

▶ Invite students to spend the day wearing blindfolds or earplugs. Have them report on their experiences and discuss how they had to modify their lifestyle to accommodate the loss.

▶ Invite students to explore ways the blind and deaf are accommodated in everyday life. Have them explore Braille on elevators and automatic teller machines. Invite students to watch TV without sound or watch closed-caption television.

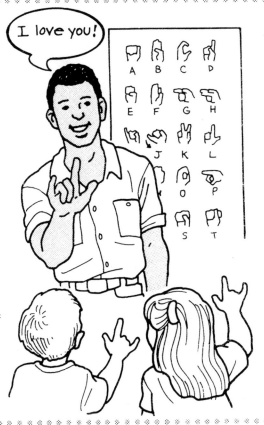

Culminating Activity

To culminate the Five Senses unit, share and reenact *Stone Soup* by Ann McGovern. Have students bring different vegetables and spices to class. Provide a ladle, large soup pot, hot plate, large stone, beef bones, butter, salt, Styrofoam cups, and spoons. Prior to reading the story, have students sit in a circle, close their eyes, and identify through smell and touch different ingredients passed to them. While reading aloud *Stone Soup*, have students close their eyes, listen, and guess which ingredients are being added to the pot. Extend the activity to include other ingredients brought in by students. After reading the story (while cooking the soup), have students write their own *Stone Soup* picture book and draw different soup ingredients. When the soup is done (2–3 hours), pour samples into cups for students to smell, taste, and enjoy.

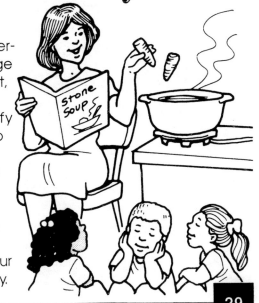

Creative Teaching Press, Inc.

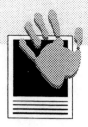

Assessment

An important goal in early childhood science education is to generate curiosity and enthusiasm about science. In a hands-on program, students should receive credit for participation and involvement as well as comprehension.

Rubric

A rubric is a scoring guide that defines student performance. Use the Performance Evaluation and Rubric (page 31) to assess student progress for each exploration.

Portfolios

Student lab sheets, journals, and self-evaluations are important parts of science portfolios. All portfolio entries should be dated so they can be chronologically compared at any time. Teacher checklists and performance evaluations can also be helpful in keeping track of progress and achievements.

Anecdotal Records

Keep written records of observations that verify students' understanding of science concepts and processes during hands-on activities. Use these to assist in student and parent conferencing.

Student Conferences

Ask students to discuss their most interesting exploration. Guide them using questions such as: *What did you learn by doing this exploration? What might you do differently if you tried it again?*

Name _____ Date _____

My Science Work

Exploration:_____

My work was:

My best!   Good.   I can do better.

By doing this exploration, I learned _____

_____

_____

If I could do it again, I would _____

_____

Performance Evaluation

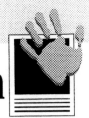

Student_____ Date _____

Check the level that best reflects student's performance.

Exploration:	Performance Level			
_____	Excellent	Very Good	Good	Needs Improvement
Shows motivation and curiosity for learning.				
Draws reasonable conclusions from science exploration.				
Demonstrates full understanding of concepts.				
Clearly communicates and listens to others.				
Accurately records and describes observations.				
Uses knowledge to solve problems or extend thinking.				

Comments:

Rubric

Excellent
Goes beyond competency, adding creativity and insight to overall performance. Shows initiative and takes charge of learning. Listens attentively to others. Shows advanced critical thinking skills. Written work is polished with detailed explanations that extend into other subject areas.

Very Good
Uses skills effectively. Listens well during discussions, contributing thoughtful ideas and opinions. Work is neat and accurate, showing evidence of higher-level thinking. Does not take risks or extend ideas into other subject areas.

Good
Shows much effort and desire to learn but is still working on mastery of skills. Written work is accurate but shows little creativity or higher-level thinking. Follows directions well but needs extra encouragement and time to organize work.

Needs Improvement
Lacks organization and effort. Student is unsure of how to use materials or uses them incorrectly. Written work is inaccurate and shows little or no creativity. Does not follow directions and needs additional guidance to perform general tasks.

Creative Teaching Press, Inc.

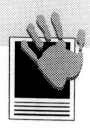

Bibliography

Children's Books

Berger, Melvin. *All about Sound*. Scholastic Inc., 1994.

Blanchard, Arlene. *Sounds My Feet Make*. Random House, 1988.

Brighton, Catherine. *My Hands, My World*. Macmillan Publishing Co., 1984.

Brown, Craig. *City Sounds*. Greenwillow Books, 1992.

Davidson, Margaret. *Helen Keller*. Scholastic Inc., 1989.

Hawkins, Colin and Jacqui. *Jungle Sounds*. Crown Publishers, Inc., 1986.

Machotka, Hana. *Breathtaking Noses*. Morrow Junior Books, 1992.

Martin, Bill Jr. and Archambault, John. *Here Are My Hands*. Henry Holt & Company, 1985.

McGovern, Ann. *Stone Soup*. Scholastic Inc., 1986.

Moncure, Jane B. *Sounds All Around*. Childrens Press, 1982.

Pallotta, Jerry. *The Spice Alphabet Book: Herbs, Spices, and Other Natural Flavors*. Charlesbridge Publishing, 1995.

Rauzon, Mark J. *Eyes and Ears, Volume 1*. William Morrow, 1994.

Showers, Paul. *Ears Are for Hearing*. HarperCollins Children's Books, 1990.

Showers, Paul. *The Listening Walk*. HarperCollins Children's Books, 1991.

Showers, Paul. *Look at Your Eyes*. HarperCollins Children's Books, 1992.

Wood, Nicholas. *Touch . . . What Do You Feel?* Troll Associates, 1991.

Worthy, Judith. *Eyes*. Doubleday, 1988.

Yolen, Jane. *Hands*. Sundance Publishers, 1976.

Resource Books

Block, J. Richard and Harold Yuker. *Can You Believe Your Eyes?* Gardner Press, 1989.

Day, Trevor. *The Random House Book of 1001 Questions and Answers about the Human Body*. Random House, 1994.

Dorling-Kindersley, Ltd. Staff. *The Visual Dictionary of the Human Body*. Dorling Kindersley, 1991.

Wollard, Kathy. *How Come?* Workman Publishing, 1993.

Creative Teaching Press, Inc.